BABY OR NOT, HERE WE GROW™

SURROGACY
THE HOSPITAL AND OTHER RELATED TOPICS

VIRGINIA L FRANK

Copyright 2025 Toku Jeve, LLC
Virginia L. Frank, Author

All Rights Reserved.
Published in the United State by More Choices Publications, a division of Toku Jeve, LLC.

Description: First Edition. Colorado: More Choices Publications, 2025.
Subjects: Non-Fiction: IVF, Surrogacy, Parenting, Children.

ISBN: 978-1-83556-399-1 Paperback
ISBN: 978-1-83556-400-4 eBook

LC ebook available at https://lccn.loc.gov/2024000803
LC record available at https://lccn.loc.gov/2024000803
Book Design by HMDPublishing.com

CONTENTS

Preparing for Baby:

A Hospital Guide for Intended Parents in Surrogacy 4

    The Legal Documents: Building Your Relationship on Paper

    Financial Information: Navigating the Costs & Insurance Post-Birth

    Planning Your Trip: Navigating the Logistics

Hospital Preparation 9

    Comfort and Care: At the Hospital

    Welcoming Baby Home: Preparing for Your Little One's Arrival

    Don't Forget Your Surrogate: Special Thoughts

    Document the Event in Pictures and Video

    Lactation Considerations for Intended Parents

    The Birth Certificate Process

    After the Birth: The Child's Story

Conclusion: 18

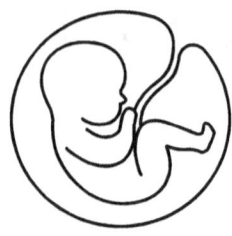

PREPARING FOR BABY: A HOSPITAL GUIDE FOR INTENDED PARENTS IN SURROGACY

Surrogacy: There isn't much written about surrogacy and what intended parents are to expect once they get closer to the birth of their child. The path hasn't been easy, but here you are on the doorstep to becoming parents! This book is your companion in preparing for a hospital stay and all those important pieces that might be missing from the puzzle. I hope that this guide helps to navigate the final steps, ensuring your hospital stay is as smooth and stress-free as possible, and allowing you to focus on what truly matters: Family.

The Legal Documents: Building Your Relationship on Paper

Before your child's birth, establishing a solid legal foundation to secure your parental rights is essential. This involves gathering all parentage, custody, or power of attorney documents from your assisted reproduction attorney and making multiple hard copies, as well as digital backups. Additionally, a hospital letter drafted by your surrogacy matching program or attorney should be sent to the hospital's social work department on the Labor and Delivery floor. This letter outlines your birth plan, legal rights, and contact information for your matching program, agency, or attorney. Attach a copy of your Pre-Birth Parentage Order signed by the Court to the letter, and ensure these documents are sent to the hospital well in advance, and bring a copy with you to the birth in case it did not make it into the surrogate's hospital records file. Alongside these legal documents, remember to bring your driver's license or passport for identification and your insurance card. If you haven't had a hospital tour already, request one in the letter to familiarize yourself and your surrogate with the hospital policies and procedures. This preparation ensures a smooth and stress-free experience during the birth of your child.

If you have not yet had an opportunity to tour the hospital, you may wish to request a tour of the OBGYN floor in this letter. This will allow you and your surrogate to become acquainted with the location, hospital policies, and expectations for the day of birth. Most surrogacy matching programs do not have a local on-the-ground social worker to meet with you and take you through the process. Therefore, you will need to be in charge of this aspect yourself and realize that you can independently schedule this tour with your surrogate. If your surrogate cannot attend the visit, consider doing the visit yourself. As intended parents, you will wish to feel comfortable with where your child will be born, and familiarize yourself with the hospital and its policies. Each hospital will have different policies and procedures, so don't forget to make a special effort for a planned visit and take notes if possible. On the day of the birth, everyone will be very excited and focused on the birth. It is best not to be disoriented when visiting a new hospital for the first time, and not knowing where to go or what is expected of you when you arrive.

Finally, create a comprehensive notification list to let everyone know about the birth. If the birth is a scheduled C-section or an induction date has been set, this notification list can be sent well in advance. This isn't just a list of people to call; it's a network of support waiting to celebrate with you. Include family, friends, colleagues, your surrogacy matching agency, and, most importantly, your attorney.

The moment your baby arrives, notify your attorney. This is critical for the timely filing of necessary legal documents, including post-birth orders, birth certificate amendments, or various surrogacy parentage decrees. Remember that each state's laws differ, so talk to your attorney before the birth so you understand the process. When writing your attorney, remember to confirm the specific information they require: the date, time, and location of birth, and, of course, your baby's name. Be aware of any legal deadlines for post-birth paperwork, if any. For international intended parents, affidavits are often required after birth to be given to your embassy, and your international attorney working on obtaining the child's citizenship in the parent's country of residence. Other items that will be required to travel back to your country of origin include, but are not limited to, passports, apostilles, and certified copies. Arrange for a notary to be on standby for you to contact after birth for these documents. The US attorney may have a traveling notary or an e-notary in their office for the convenience of the intended parents and the surrogacy process. These small details can make a big difference in ensuring a smooth legal process and peace of mind. Lastly, if a translation of the document is needed, please research in advance who to contact for a certified translator. Your international surrogacy attorney should be able to help point you in the right direction, so always stay in touch.

Financial Information: Navigating the Costs & Insurance Post-Birth

The Child: Intended parents are ultimately responsible for all medical bills and care related to the baby after birth. In the United States, U.S. citizens can typically add their child to their health insurance policy immediately after birth. Contacting your insurance provider to initiate this process is essential. If you are an international intended parent, you must purchase a child's medical policy in order to have medical bills covered after birth. Paying out of pocket is always an option, but be aware that if the child were to go into the NICU, the medical costs could be astronomical, and you would be responsible for payment of those bills. Please remember to check with your insurance broker about purchasing a child's health insurance policy early in the pregnancy.

Additionally, a visit to the hospital's business office is necessary to provide your insurance information or arrange cash payment for the child's stay. If you have a planned C-section or an induction, you could plan to visit the hospital a day or so early to get all insurance information in the surrogate's medical file and hospital records. Various medical providers will need to be given insurance and billing information after birth; These providers include all well-baby checks, tests, and vaccinations administered by the hospital. In cases where the child requires care in the NICU due to medical issues, an extended stay, or prematurity of the baby, the intended parents are responsible for those expenses. It's highly recommended that intended parents confirm with their current healthcare provider the procedures for adding their newborn to their policy. Once this is established, you will be responsible for any co-pays and deductibles associated with the birth. Intended parents without existing insurance should begin investigating options for purchasing child health insurance early in the surrogacy journey, as going without coverage is strongly discouraged. Proactive planning is paramount to ensure the health and well-being of the newborn.

The Surrogate: When talking about the responsibility of the intended parents for surrogates' medical bills, intended parents bear the ultimate responsibility for all the surrogate's medical expenses related to the surrogacy pregnancy. These financial obligations are comprehensively detailed within the gestational carrier agreement, which was signed before the embryo transfer. To ensure seamless payment processing, the surrogate should direct all co-pays, deductibles, and other medical bills to the designated surrogacy escrow company whenever possible. Keep in mind that the gestational surrogate may receive medical bills after the birth at her home for six (6) months or more after birth. These medical bills should be given to the surrogacy escrow company, which acts as a neutral third party and will manage the disbursement of funds to the hospital or medical providers, adhering strictly to the stipulations outlined in the gestational carrier agreement. This system streamlines payments and provides consistency for all parties involved. Be certain to check with your matching program and your surrogate to ensure these medical bills do not go unpaid or to collections under the surrogate's name. Remember that after birth, someone should monitor if all the birth medical bills are forwarded to the Escrow account after birth. Intended parents might consider purchasing health insurance monitoring services to ensure all premiums are paid on time.

Planning Your Trip: Navigating the Logistics

If you are traveling, consider renting a suite or a home for more space and kitchen facilities. Check for online discounts before booking a hotel. Call ahead to confirm if the hotel provides travel cribs or bassinets. If completing a surrogacy within your state, you can typically leave once the baby is discharged. Confirm with your agency or attorney if any legal circumstances require a longer stay. Arrange an appointment for your baby's check-up within three days of discharge. The airline may require a medical release if you are flying home with a newborn under two weeks old. You should check with the airlines on their specific requirements. By preparing in advance and considering all these details, you can ensure a smoother and more joyful experience as you welcome your baby into your family. This is more than about packing a bag. It's about preparing for a new chapter filled with love, laughter, and the extraordinary miracle of parenthood. Safe travels and best wishes on your journey!

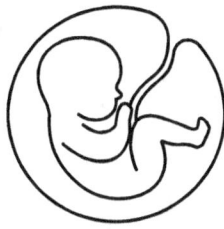

HOSPITAL PREPARATION

Comfort and Care: At the Hospital

While the birth of the baby is paramount, remember that you too, need care and comfort during this experience. The ideas below should help in preparing to pack your bag for your hospital stay. This will prioritize your well-being during this emotionally and physically demanding time.

It is essential to understand hospital accommodations. Hospitals prioritize the birthing surrogate's needs and sleeping arrangements first. For intended parents, accommodations may be limited depending on the hospital and how many births are occurring at the time of your visit. At times, there may be no rooms available for intended parents to spend time alone with their child. However, as rooms and availability change, it may be possible to ask if you can have your own room for bonding and giving the gestational carrier some private time. Regardless of the situation, always be respectful of hospital staff and their procedures. They are there to support everyone involved.

Packing layers of comfortable clothing is highly recommended, as hospitals can be surprisingly cold. Comfortable shoes or slippers are a must for all the walking you'll be doing. Always prepare for a potentially longer stay than anticipated by packing enough clothing. If overnight stays are possible, pack pajamas, your own pillow, and a blanket for added comfort. Leave these items in your car until you confirm whether a room is available. Don't bring them into the Labor and Delivery area initially.

Remember your medications – both prescription and over-the-counter. Labor and childbirth can be a long process, so pack entertainment items like books, magazines, an iPad, a Kindle, headphones, or games to keep yourself occupied. A toiletry bag with essentials is a must. Don't forget the small things that make a difference: a toothbrush, toothpaste, shampoo, soap, deodorant, makeup, and any other personal care items. Staying hydrated is crucial. Bring a refillable water bottle. Many hospitals have water refill stations.

Pack a front-button shirt for each parent for skin-to-skin contact with the baby. Many fathers will want to have skin-to-skin contact as well. Consider shopping for a shirt designed for this purpose. Bring your camera and charger if you want to capture high-quality photos or videos. Be mindful of hospital policies regarding photography and videography. Pack some non-perishable snacks like protein bars, fruit bars, or nuts to keep you going. Hospital cafeterias may have limited hours. Consider meal options in advance. Will you rely on the hospital cafeteria, nearby restaurants, or food delivery services? Download the apps for these services before the big day!

Decide whether you will use the hospital's pediatrician to assess your child's health after birth or contact your own pediatrician and let them know of your child's birth. Make sure you let the hospital know of your choice in pediatricians and that they will need to contact him or her once the child is born. This should be done in advance of the birth. Lastly, newborns need a check-up within a few days of birth to check on the baby's weight and eating habits. Schedule this appointment with the pediatrician's office once the child is born.

Lastly, if you have any special keepsake items you want to include in photos or keep as mementos, bring them with you. Many intended parents want to record their feelings and thoughts during the process and at the hospital. If you are one of those parents, don't forget to bring along the journal to record your thoughts and gratitude at the hospital.

Welcoming Baby Home: Preparing for Your Little One's Arrival

Your baby will need some essentials as well. Pack at least two going-home outfits in both newborn and preemie sizes, as you may not know the baby's exact size upon birth. Wash all baby clothes before packing them to remove any chemicals from new fabrics. This list includes socks, gowns, and booties. Pack at least two (2) blankets of varying thickness for different temperatures. If you are not heading home immediately, bring a travel crib, crib sheets, a changing pad, and any other necessary sleeping items. If traveling from afar, you might consider purchasing some of these items locally to avoid packing them. Bring a few pacifiers, even if you don't plan to use them regularly, and a small tube of diaper cream. Remember, a properly installed, hospital-approved car seat is mandatory for hospital discharge. Ensure you know how to install it correctly. Bring your preferred brand if you plan to use a formula, as hospitals may only stock certain types. Lastly, research and bring with you the sterilized bottles and nipples of your choice. There are many to choose from in the marketplace, so research these choices before the birth.

Don't Forget Your Surrogate: Special Thoughts

In all of the excitement about the new baby, intended parents may overlook a celebration of the surrogate and her contribution and sacrifice for the life she brought into this world for you. A special gift at the hospital can be very appreciated as she is now a part of your life journey. First, always bring flowers and a special handwritten card to show your thoughts about her and her sacrifice for you. A handwritten letter can be a wonderful keepsake for years to come for a surrogate. Other pre-planned options to consider are customized gifts with her initials or her name on a special item. Many intended parents may also give a photo album to save pictures of the special, memorable moments during the pregnancy, at delivery, or with other members of your family. Of course, no one likes hospital food, and a healthy birth hospital stay is between twenty-four and forty-eight hours. Finally, figure out your surrogate's favorite food or meal and bring that to her and her partner, friends, or other children when at the hospital before discharge. Lastly, consider capturing the pictures and videos of the birth to remember the once-in-a-lifetime event.

Document the Event in Pictures and Video

Special moments should be saved, and it is great to present the moments with videos and pictures. With today's smartphones, you can easily capture moments to be viewed for a lifetime. However, many intended parents decided to have a special video camera of their own or bring a professional into the hospital after the birth of the child to get those once-in-a-lifetime moments on tape. Special "first" pictures of the child can also be completed through professional photography services. Whatever you decide is right for you, don't forget to document the moment. This time will never come again!

Lactation Considerations for Intended Parents

The journey to parenthood through surrogacy is often filled with unique considerations, and feeding your little one is a central part of that experience. While the surrogate carried and delivered the baby, intended parents who did not give birth can still explore the possibility of inducing lactation. This process allows some parents to experience the special bond of breastfeeding and provide their baby with the incredible benefits of breast milk. It's essential, however, to approach this path with realistic expectations. Induced lactation is different from lactation after a pregnancy. The body hasn't experienced the hormonal shifts of gestation, and therefore, it may not produce a full milk supply. It requires significant commitment, effort, and a deep understanding of the process. The cornerstone of successful induced lactation lies in professional guidance. Consulting an IBCLC is essential. Think of them as your personal coach and cheerleader throughout this journey.

A lactation consultant can provide personalized guidance and support, assess your individual circumstances, and develop a plan tailored to your specific needs. They can help you navigate the complexities of pumping techniques, address any concerns that may arise, and offer invaluable emotional support. They are your go-to resource for navigating this unique path. For some intended parents, certain medications, under the close guidance of a physician, can help stimulate milk production. These medications work by mimicking the hormonal changes associated with pregnancy. Discussing these options thoroughly with your doctor and carefully weighing the potential benefits against any possible side effects is crucial. This is a decision that should be made in conjunction with your healthcare provider, ensuring your overall well-being.

Frequent and consistent pumping is the engine that drives milk production in induced lactation. Think of it as sending constant signals to your body that milk is needed. A hospital-grade pump is often recommended due to its efficiency and ability to mimic the sucking action of a baby. Your lactation consultant can help you establish a pumping schedule that optimizes milk production while fitting into your lifestyle. This will likely involve pumping multiple times a day, even when you don't feel like it. Consistency is key. As you begin your lactation journey, a Supplemental Nursing System (SNS) can be a valuable tool. A Supplemental Nursing System is a device that allows supplemental formula or donor milk to be provided to the baby while they are nursing at the breast. This serves two important purposes: it ensures the baby receives adequate nutrition while simultaneously stimulating the breast and encouraging continued milk production. Furthermore, it fosters the crucial bonding experience of breastfeeding, even before a full milk supply is established.

The world of galactagogues – foods, herbs, and supplements believed to support milk production – is often explored by parents pursuing induced lactation. From fenugreek to oatmeal, there's a wide array of options to consider. However, it's vital to research these options thoroughly and discuss them with your doctor or lactation consultant. While some galactagogues may be helpful, others may have potential side effects or interact with medications. A cautious and informed approach is always best. Perhaps the most underestimated aspect of induced lactation is the emotional support required. It can be a challenging and sometimes frustrating process. There will be days when you feel discouraged and question whether it's all worth it. Having a strong support system – your partner, your IBCLC, and other parents who have gone through similar experiences – is essential. Remember that every drop of breast milk you provide your baby is a gift, and celebrate every milestone, no matter how small. This journey is a testament to your love and dedication; you are not alone.

Therefore, if you plan to induce lactation, pack a breast pump, nursing bra, supplemental nursing system, nipple cream, and breast pads. If you plan to pump and store milk, ask the hospital about their refrigeration facilities, as they will probably store the milk for you while you are at the hospital.

The Birth Certificate Process

Another essential item to consider after the birth of your child is the process of obtaining the child's birth certificate at the State of Birth's Department of Health and Environment (also known as Vital Records). Many intended parents assume that this is an automatic process completed by the hospital after you provide them with documentation of parentage. However, the hospital only collects information and does not issue birth certificates.

The Vital Records department in each state keeps track of births and deaths and will issue birth certificates for each child's birth. Likewise, each state has various forms that they would like completed by the birthing surrogate and intended parents. Therefore, the hospital must send all information and proof of parentage to Vital Records after the birth. Since the surrogate has given birth to the child, her name may be initially listed as a parent, and your name will be substituted after the documentation of parentage is given to the State Vital Records department through the proper channel. Please visit the birth certificate clerk at the birthing hospital to fill out important information regarding the surrogacy birth. Make sure to have a copy of your pre-birth parentage order to provide to the birth certificate hospital clerk. It is possible that the hospital may not be familiar with surrogacy births and might not be able to answer questions regarding the modification of the child's birth certificate. Please talk to your surrogacy attorney regarding the process in advance to understand what to expect. Your attorney will guide you through the required documentation. There are many steps for amending the birth certificate, and these vary significantly by state. Competent legal counsel is indispensable for this process.

After the Birth: The Child's Story

Many intended parents struggle with ideas on explaining their own story to their children. Scrapbooking or online companies that print books for you of your experience offer a wonderful opportunity for families to personalize their surrogacy journey and create a lasting keepsake. Unlike traditional baby books, scrapbooks allow you to continue adding pages as your child grows and their story unfolds. Here are some helpful tips for creating a meaningful surrogacy journey scrapbook:

1. **Start Early**: Begin assembling the scrapbook as soon as you get matched with a surrogate, after your child's arrival, or even during the surrogacy journey. Label photos promptly to ensure you capture details while they're fresh in your memory.

2. **Maintain an Authentic Voice**: Tell the story from your own perspective without projecting feelings onto your child. While the scrapbook pages remain unchanged, your child's understanding and perception will evolve over time.

3. **Share Personal Reflections**: Document your emotions throughout the surrogacy journey to show your child how eagerly awaited their birth. After the child arrives, jot down notes ranging from daily routines to deep personal reflections. Keep notes or a journal called **Our Family's Surrogacy Journey Insights**: If possible, gather information about your child's surrogate and extended family during the surrogacy process and at the hospital. Ask questions that your child might want answers to in the future.

4. **Highlight the Surrogate Family Connections**: Consider dedicating a section of the scrapbook to your child's surrogate family in open surrogacy arrangements. Encourage them to contribute by sharing details about themselves, akin to the Family Favorites section in your Surrogate Journey's Family Profile. Think about

all the questions you might have if you were born via a surrogate, and write those questions down to ask your surrogate.

5. **Duplicate Sent Communications**: If you have been sending letters or pictures to your child's surrogate, include copies in the scrapbook. This demonstrates that the relationship remains open and showcases milestones shared with the birth family. Any type of ultrasound pictures or "firsts" that were shared by your surrogate with you through texts, video, or email can be included in the scrapbook.

6. **Be Transparent and Age-Appropriate**: The more your child knows, the less uncertainty they face, aiding their identity formation as they grow. Children who know and understand their surrogacy journey from a young age are less likely to be shocked and surprised later in life. Keep explanations age-appropriate and expand on them as your child's understanding and questions mature. Therefore, some ideas and concepts can be introduced through pictures early on and become a commonplace discussion as the child grows. If you used an egg, sperm, or donated embryo, explain this in age-appropriate ways so that the child doesn't discover it later inadvertently and wonder why it was a secret. Having an open, honest, age-appropriate story with your child will ensure a happy and honest relationship with them as they grow.

7. **Include Milestones and Mementos**: Capture essential events such as your child's birth, court parentage/adoption orders, dates or documents to include, and coming home. Explain your reasons for doing surrogacy and the origins of your child's name. Use mementos like footprints, Pre and Post Birth Orders, and maps showing your journey to your child.

8. **Preserve the Original**: Make color copies of the scrapbook so your child can have their own to handle while preserving the original. You can do this yourself with scrapbooking material or use an online site that can put together a book for you once you update the pictures and information. Sites such as Scrapbook.com, Creative Memories, Hero Arts & Spellbinder might be options for those who don't have time or ability to make a book themselves.

9. **Engage with the scrapbook together**: Regularly look through the scrapbook with your child until they can read it independently. Little kids like to flip through the book to view their story. Allow them to share it with others, but don't impose it upon them.

By following these tips, you can create a beautiful and personal scrapbook that will serve as a cherished reminder of your family's unique and loving journey.

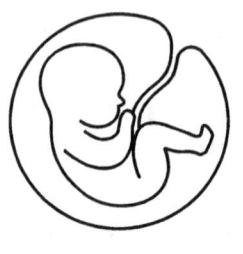

CONCLUSION:

This comprehensive guide has equipped you with the knowledge and tools to navigate your surrogacy hospital stay with confidence. From the essential legal documentation to the comforting details of personal care, each aspect has been addressed to empower you on this remarkable journey. Remember that this is a celebration of family, a testament to the power of love and the miracle of new life. While the logistics and preparations are essential, the proper focus remains on the precious moments you will share with your child. Embrace the joy, cherish the memories, and allow yourself to be fully present as you embark on this incredible adventure of parenthood. Welcome, little one. Your family awaits.

For an even more in-depth exploration of the entire surrogacy process, be sure to check our Surrogacy Journal: Baby or Not Here We Grow... This comprehensive guide empowers intended parents with the knowledge, tools, and resources to confidently navigate the surrogacy journey. From understanding the basics of surrogacy to preparing for your baby's arrival, the guide covers every step of the process. You can find it soon on the Barnes and Noble website and Amazon. If you are interested in an IVF Journal or a US Private Adoption Informational Journal, you can also find those on Barnes and Noble and Amazon under *Baby or Not Here We Grow* as well.

Disclaimer: This content is provided for informational purposes only and is not intended as legal or medical advice. Reading or interacting with this material does not establish legal or medical advice.

CONCLUSION:

Laws and regulations vary widely by jurisdiction and can change frequently; thus, readers should always consult with a qualified attorney or legal advisor for specific advice tailored to their individual circumstances before taking any action based on this information. It is imperative to seek the counsel of a qualified healthcare provider for any medical guidance pertaining to the surrogacy procedure or lactation.